Rod Tobin's experience in dealing with male sexual abuse is evident in this timely, concise and clear exposition of treatment strategies designed for male survivors. A must for survivors, spouses and therapists.

Patrick Beausang, M.Ed.
Clinical member, American
Association of Marriage and
Family Therapy

Rod Tobin has become an expert on treatment of male sexual abuse without losing his compassion for survivors. This model addresses the differences between male and female survivor issues in an effective and respectful way. IT WORKS!

Alice Schmidt-Hanbidge,
MSW, CSW

Alone and Forgotten *represents a tremendous contribution, not only to the professional therapeutic community, but also to the employer community and general public. If you are an employer, manager, spouse or survivor, I know this book will bring to you comfort and understanding of this very difficult subject.*

Mark Schneider
Manager, Human Resources
MTD Products Limited

Alone & Forgotten: The Sexually Abused Man

Rod Tobin

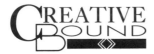

Books that Inspire, Help and Heal

Published by Creative Bound Inc.
Box 424, Carp, Ontario
Canada K0A 1L0
(613) 831-3641

ISBN 0-921165-60-9
Printed and bound in Canada

Book design by Wendelina O'Keefe

Cover image © Photodisc

Canadian Cataloguing in Publication Data

Tobin, Rod
    Alone & forgotten : the sexually abused man

Includes bibliographical references.
ISBN 0-921165-60-9

    1. Abused men--Rehabilitation. 2. Adult child sexual abuse victims. 3. Sexual abuse victims. I. Title. II. Title: Alone and forgotten.

HV6570.T62 1999   362.8'081   C99-900379-8

Preface

This book describes the major symptoms of sexually abused men—anger, mistrust and meaninglessness—and some ways in which the healing process may be enhanced. We explore the cause of these symptoms and discuss the therapeutic process. The problem of early dropout is addressed, and suggestions are given for ways to minimize risk of relapse.

The two predominant models of therapy used in this book are a psychoanalytic approach and a behavioral, solution-focused approach.

Chapter 1 uses a psychoanalytic approach. Much of the work done early in my career was based on psychoanalysis. My consequent familiarity with unconscious defenses proved invaluable when explaining to clients just how they developed unhealthy patterns that impair personal functioning. Such explanation is not always a part of therapy; however, in the case of sexually abused men it was useful. It allowed them to overcome a long-standing belief that they were victims of their own weaknesses and that change was impossible.

Chapters 2, 3 and 4 employ behavioral approaches to recovery, and present my final treatment methods, which were influenced by a solution-focused approach to recovery.

My approach does not include some issues that are frequently the subject of therapy. These issues include confusion about sexual identity, survivors who are perpetrators, and drug or alcohol abuse. It has been my experience that these issues are too overwhelming to confront early in treatment and may be responsible for early dropout if confronted directly and at an early stage. In fact, sexually abused men are more receptive to the idea of tackling anger, mistrust and meaninglessness early in the treatment and are then in a better position to deal with other serious issues.

Chapter 5 presents an overview of the therapeutic process that can serve to move a survivor toward recovery.

For approximately five years, I had worked with sexually abused women. As I began to work with male survivors, and listened to their experiences, it became apparent that there are no established effective treatment models for male survivors, as there are for females. It seemed necessary to develop something that would work. The therapeutic models that I have come to use really unfolded as my clients provided input over a four-year period. The issues that are the focus of treatment reflect the clients' priorities, not mine.

Some therapists may disagree with the order of treatment, or with the strategy of omitting certain issues in the first stages of treatment. I have attempted to follow the injunction of solution-focused therapy that states that the agenda should be that of the client and not the therapist.

This book is intended to be used either as an aid to therapists who are working with male survivors or as a tool for male survivors themselves who are working toward recovery. Either way, I hope my work is helpful in overcoming the devastation that results from the sexual abuse of young men and, if this is untreated, persists into adulthood.

Contents

Introduction

"Why should I feel guilty? That bastard should be drawn and quartered. I didn't do anything wrong."

"How would you feel if some dirty old creep put his thing in you? Try to imagine how you would feel."

"I don't give a damn if I get compensation or not. I just want him punished. There is nothing bad enough you could do to him as far as I'm concerned."

In 1992, I began working with men who had been sexually abused in a boys' training school. These men now range in age from their late 20s to 65, the age of my oldest client. Initially, I used the models of treatment with which I was familiar. However, I quickly learned that male sexually abused clients did not respond favorably to the process of treatment that proved to be so effective for female abuse victims. In fact, the word "victim" was not well received by male clients.

When I began working with these men, the first few clients

dropped out very quickly, and I knew that nothing constructive had happened. At that point I consulted other therapists, as well as books and other materials, but failed to find any workable approach to treatment.

I called the men who had left therapy and asked them to come back and talk to me. When they did, I told them that in spite of my experience and success with abused women, I was obviously having no success with them. I told them that I didn't know what I could do to be helpful.

They agreed with me. "We know you don't know—nobody knows. That's why we're ignored." I asked them if they would work with me to help develop something that would work and they agreed. Since they were all "pissed off," we began by working with anger.

It is not the purpose of this book to pass judgment on our society or my colleagues. However, it has been with much distress that I have listened to the experiences sexually abused men have suffered at the hands of others. The three main reasons that sexually abused men fail to disclose and avoid seeking treatment are these:

1. negative judgment by family members and loss of friendship

2. stigma in the eyes of society

3. lack of understanding by therapists and unpleasant experiences in therapeutic settings

There is no simple way to eliminate these three factors. It is because they are so significant that I was determined to explore further the plight of these men and endeavor to establish a workable treatment model that could lead to recovery. With their assistance, I believe this has been achieved.

There can be no better source for solutions than the clients themselves. Because my clients decided to bear with me in the therapeutic setting, I am now able to record their experiences and ways in which they successfully overcame symptoms that impaired their well-being.

Chapters 2, 3 and 4 focus on the three main symptoms suffered by male sexual-abuse survivors. Often these symptoms result from emotions that lie beneath the surface and remain unexpressed. These three symptoms are anger, mistrust and meaninglessness. They give rise to broken relationships, dissatisfaction with jobs and work-related endeavors, withdrawal from other people, depression, low self-esteem, substance abuse and even suicide. While men can become very closed about certain issues, such as guilt/shame, sexuality and low self-esteem, they are approachable on the subjects of anger, mistrust and meaninglessness, and they can deal with these issues early in the treatment process. They will discuss these issues in detail, and without exception they have shown remarkable ability to achieve change in the direction of better functioning.

Chapter 5 presents a description of the therapeutic process as a positive experience and highlights such subjects as the dynamics of the client-therapist relationship, disclosure of abuse, and potential relapse.

By now you are probably asking, "What happened to Chapter 1?" I wished to describe the symptoms that sexually abused men experience so that I could describe the reason such symptoms exist. These symptoms are not accidental. Underlying the symptoms of anger, mistrust and meaninglessness are particular defenses. The strongest of these are unconscious repression and conscious suppression.

As a rule, I do not go through the process of discussing defenses at length with my clients, but sexually abused men are exceptions. It is because of their extremely favorable response to an understanding of defenses that I have felt compelled to make it part of the treatment itself. Perhaps this knowledge is so appealing to men because it separates them from their problem areas by revealing a partly unconscious process over which they have little control. In other words, they come to realize that behaviors that they themselves do not particularly like are explainable, and can be changed. A non-judgmental attitude, coupled with a distanced approach they can identify with, gives them hope.

Chapter 1, then, discusses the defenses employed by sexually abused men, especially repression and suppression. The recognition and discussion of these defenses are vital to treatment because, in my experience, these men come to therapy believing that they simply are who they are and can never change.

Men who are survivors of sexual abuse have two fundamental qualities that can lead to recovery. One, they wish to change. Two, they possess the courage to do so. I have witnessed these qualities during therapy and have seen remarkable changes take place as a result. Perhaps it is time that others gain more understanding of what these men need. I cannot help but think that more men would come forward if they knew they would be treated by all segments of society with sound knowledge and given the respect that they deserve.

Chapter 1

Defenses

Defenses are part of the repertoire of mechanisms that protect us from anxiety by keeping intolerable or unacccptable impulses or threats from conscious awareness. The concept of defense is rooted in classical psychoanalytic theory.

Defenses operate unconsciously. For example, a man who is very angry with his wife for not coming home on time may find himself extremely irritated with the gas station attendant who keeps him waiting. His anger has been redirected to another object, which permits expression of the impulse in an insignificant, non-threatening situation rather than in a situation that risks significant conflict. This shifting of feelings or conflicts at an unconscious level is called **displacement**.

Defenses are not to be confused with coping mechanisms. Defenses operate outside of conscious awareness, while coping mechanisms are used deliberately. T.C. Kroeber describes the differences.

1. Defenses cannot be used deliberately, while coping mechanisms can.

2. Defenses are rigid, compelled and perhaps conditioned, whereas coping mechanisms are flexible, purposive and involve choice.

3. Defenses are pushed by the past rather than pulled by the future.

4. Defenses distort the present situation rather than being oriented to the reality requirements of the present situation.

5. Defenses operate as if it were necessary and possible wholly to remove disturbing feelings and may involve unrealistic "magical thinking" rather than operating in accordance with reality.

6. Defenses allow impulse gratification only through suffrage (suffering or pain) rather than allowing impulse satisfaction in an open, ordered and tempered way. For example, an insecure man who is convinced his wife will leave him for a better man may bring about that very occurrence through persistent negative behavior.

All people use defenses, but their exact type and extent vary from individual to individual. Defenses falsify and distort reality to some extent, although in individuals who function effectively such distortions are minimal and do not impair healthy functioning. To the degree that such defenses enable the person to function optimally without undue anxiety, they are considered to be effective.

In many instances, however, depending on the intensity of the conflict, the nature of the current stimuli evoking it, or the fragility or pervasiveness of the defense itself, such mechanisms may prove to be ineffective, or maladaptive. They may (1) prevent the individual from gaining needed satisfaction—such as acceptance, sense of accomplishment, sense of worth or sense of security; (2) be insufficient to contain the anxiety or conflict so that the person becomes overwhelmed, symptomatic or disorganized; or (3) distort reality to such a degree that the sense of self is impaired.

A complicating factor in evaluating defenses is that they can have both adaptive and maladaptive effects within the same individual. For example, a recovered alcoholic's ability to defend against experiencing certain emotions that might weaken his ability to remain sober may be adaptive. Such a defense, however, may also limit the degree to which he can experience and verbalize anger or participate in and enjoy intimacy with a spouse.

Efforts directed toward modifying defenses create anxiety and often are resisted by the individual. Such resistance operates unconsciously. The person does not seek deliberately to maintain his or her defenses. The resistance, however, creates obstacles to achieving the very changes that the person says he or she would like. A shy individual who wants to improve his relations with others by becoming more assertive and outgoing may change the subject when it is suggested that there are social activities in which he or she might engage in order to meet new friends. Such an individual may seem uncooperative or disinterested, when in actuality the topic makes him quite anxious, as it threatens his characteristic mode of defense.

Significant others or a therapist may wish to try to lessen or modify certain maladaptive defenses in a given individual because they interfere with effective coping. However, such mechanisms also serve as an important protective function for the person. Chess and Thomas state that in situations that are excessively stressful it would appear that the use of defense mechanisms is necessary to organize the strengths and capacities needed for success. For example, intense anger may be held and later redirected, or displaced, from the provoker onto another object, as we saw earlier in this chapter. This permits expression of the impulse in a less significant, non-destructive situation.

In some instances a defense mechanism may prove to be less adaptive. A person may deny the symptoms of a serious illness because of fear and thus not seek medical attention. The outcome could prove fatal.

Defenses are evident in everyday life. The behavior that results from them allows therapists to observe and explore indications of internal conflict, and interpret their meaning to the survivor. At this point, insight by the survivor and the therapist becomes part of the treatment. It is important to note, however, that insight alone does not provide correction of maladaptive behavior. Rather, insight may lead to exploration of measures necessary to achieve the desired state.

Defenses and Sexually Abused Men

Sexually abused males are constantly wondering about their maladaptive state. Perhaps the feeling of being out of control, the lack of understanding of failures in relationships, the feeling of constant underlying anger or the inability to complete life's goals act as catalysts to gain insight into behavior. Such feelings may be viewed as signals that there are unconscious, or partially unconscious, forces at work, which impair fulfillment of life's goals.

In the case of sexually abused men, the unconscious force that proves to be most damaging is **repression**. Repression can be defined as the unconscious exclusion of memories or feelings from awareness. Repression is not under voluntary control. It represents an unconscious defense against threat.

Repression's conscious counterpart is **suppression**—a deliberate effort to block an impulse or feeling.

In my practice, I go to great lengths to distinguish whether a person is using conscious or unconscious forces. Often repression and suppression are intimate partners in directing a person's attempts to cope with reality. It is valuable to recognize the separateness of these forces: suppression may represent a one-time effort to hide one's true feelings, while repression is an ongoing unconscious process. Repression can become a habitual response to stressful situations and, as such, requires ongoing expenditure of emotional energy. An unending cycle of defending oneself against irrational threats may ensue and consume immeasurable amounts of energy.

One of my clients, a very distraught young man, displayed both protective mechanisms. The following excerpts from an interview demonstrate these mechanisms at work. The client suppresses feelings in present situations, while giving evidence of ongoing repression.

> Client: *"I can't believe it. I blew more relationships than I can even talk about. And here I am, thinking about how I can get my best friend's wife in bed."*

> Therapist: *"Are these serious thoughts or just passing whims?"*

Client: "I'm really attracted to her. The other night, I almost asked her if she was interested in me."

Therapist: "But you didn't ask."

Client: "I almost did. But I don't have that many friends. I just couldn't betray a buddy. As much as I wanted to, I had to swallow that shit and put it out of my mind."

Excerpt from the same interview:

Client: "I remember the night that bastard came into my room. I can still see his shadow standing there in the dark, taking off his clothes."

Therapist: "What were you feeling at the time?"

Client: "I don't know. I guess I should have been feeling scared or pissed off: here it comes again."

Therapist: "Do you want to go on?"

Client: "Sure. He got on top of me and I can still remember everything he did. I closed my eyes until he went away."

Therapist: "So, you remember everything that happened."

Client: "Yes, I'm getting angry thinking about it. It wasn't the first time he did that. I still hate the look of him. If I could see him now I'd probably kill him."

Therapist: "What do you see when you remember that scene?"

Client: "I can see the room. My stuffed bear is on the dresser. There are lots of shadows on the wall; you know, the leaves on the trees outside. I'll never forget how big he looked to me then. He spoke so softly, like he was my friend and I should trust him."

Therapist: "I'm really impressed with your memory of those details. I can't imagine how you must have felt while this was going on."

Client: "Who knows? How would you feel? I guess I was scared."

Therapist: "Is that how you felt at the time?"

Client: "I suppose so."

Therapist: "I want you to give me your best effort to describe your feelings at the time."

Client: "I don't know. I remember the whole scene but I just don't know what I was feeling. I guess I went numb. I just don't recall."

In the first excerpt, the client was blocking an impulse in a conscious, deliberate way. He reports hiding his true feelings to prevent anxiety and guilt. The betrayal of his best friend represents a threatening event. This is suppression at work.

But what is happening when a person can so vividly recall details of a traumatic event, yet is unable to recall feelings that accompanied the event? Repression has protected against intolerance of the harsh reality, not only in the past, but for years thereafter. If you suggested to the man in the interview that he deliberately forgot his feelings associated with the abuse, you would witness an intense denial. You would learn a quick lesson in the difference between repression and suppression.

The strength of repression in the abused male is significant in comparison with the abused female. There is little doubt that repression substantially reduces the spectrum of emotions by blocking the ability to feel appropriate emotions. Within our culture men are taught to avoid such feelings as guilt, shame and depression—feelings that women commonly deal with in therapy. Men are not so inclined to be open about such feelings. However, feelings such as love, affection and trust are readily discussed by men, especially the absence of these feelings and the difficulty of exhibiting them in an ongoing way.

Th abused male may experience hurt, embarrassment, confusion and pleasure during the abusive event as intolerable emotions. The repression of such emotions may lead to present difficulties in displaying love, affection and trust because these feelings may be associated with old responses (hurt, embarrassment, etc.) that need to be defended against.

Let us examine the original responses, at the time of the abuse, that may bring on defenses today because of perceived threat.

Hurt

Hurt is the result of disappointment of our expectations of others. We expect persons in a position of trust to act accordingly, and they may cause hurt by violation of that trust. A young male feels trust, love and respect for a significant other and expects protection from that person; suddenly those feelings are made conditional upon sexual favors. The young man, rather than being accepted as a person, has been used sexually. The result is intense hurt—a hurt so unacceptable that the person's ego is damaged; anxiety, self-doubt and a sense of loss become overwhelming. To add to the intensity of the hurt, there is no one to help the young person deal with the feeling, as the adult can threaten or manipulate the abused into maintaining secrecy.

A ten-year-old who is rejected by his friends and falls into despair could expect to be consoled by caring parents. He would regain a sense of self and learn something about social skills. A sexually abused boy, on the other hand, must act of his own accord. He must rely on underdeveloped judgment and coping skills. He must establish protection from his anxiety, and such protection takes the form of repression. Thus, life goes on. The hurt seems to disappear, at least at the conscious level.

But the cycle of hurt and repression has begun. Perception of hurt becomes associated with significant others in intimate situations or with authority figures, or with any situation related to the original event. A feeling of great vulnerability results, and this hurt and vulnerability are repressed. So the next time a hurtful situation is perceived, the hurt is even greater, and *it* must be repressed. And the cycle continues.

Embarrassment

The young male has limited knowledge about sexuality and mixed responses to it. Masturbation provides pleasurable sensations and relief of his sexual impulses. Sexual fantasy plays a major role in his life. Usually such fantasy is targeted at intercourse with female recipients. Later, fantasy gives way to fact, and the young male participates in the act of sex. This is likely to lead to a complex mixture of thoughts and emotions, including primitive thoughts of love and commitment, pride in prowess, desire for acceptance by others, or guilt and shame. The young male may gain acceptance by peers through sharing of the conquest, or he may receive a negative reaction from parents, teachers or other authority figures. Consequently, he may be uncertain as to whether he should feel pride or shame.

Usually an abused male is a victim of seduction by an older person. In the normal course of development, as we have seen, a mixture of emotions is inevitable. But in the case of the abused male the conflict of feelings is extreme to the point of being traumatic. To comprehend the extremities of feelings, we might try to imagine a young male describing his sexual experience with an older male to his peer group. This image gives new meaning to the concept of embarrassment.

Yet an abused male must relate such experiences to his internal self, and cope with internal dialogue. This process may prove to be far too overwhelming at the feeling level. The fact that the abused at a later date can recall the event, but not the embarrassment of the trauma, shows that repression is operating as a means to face tomorrow. For all intents and purposes, the abused has managed to internalize the event and, at the same time, defend the ego against the embarrassment of the intense feelings aroused at the time they occurred.

Please note that I have used the term embarrassment rather than guilt/shame. The feelings of guilt and shame have proven to be unacceptable to men during therapeutic sessions, and broaching them could impair the therapeutic relationship.

Confusion

Confusion occurs when a person is unable to explain how his or her physical or emotional being fits into his or her environment. Confusion produces anxiety about the unknown.

Sexuality, as a part of our developmental growth, can become a source of pleasure and expression of love if it follows its natural path leading to adulthood. During pivotal stages of growth, the interruption of sexual curiosity may lead to serious, difficult questions about sexual identity. Sexual abuse by an older person may produce conflicting emotions such as love–hate, pleasure–pain, need to share and secrecy. Such conflict results in confusion.

When the abused is unable to understand intense conflict surrounding sexuality, he needs to find immediate resolution of the conflict in order to have the emotional energy to devote to other developmental needs. Abused females find such immediate relief in disassociation, a defense that prohibits recall of the event and the feelings around it. With the male victim, repression is more predominant. Perhaps disassociation would damage the male ego beyond repair, because the male is conditioned to believe that problems should be faced and dealt with. Therefore, to him, repression is a compromise. If he represses the negative feelings associated with the sexual event, the male can, as he is taught to do, look the event in the eye without the resultant intolerable feelings.

Pleasure

As a simple working definition, pleasure may be considered any feeling associated with joy or happiness. While it would seem reasonable to repress negative feelings, why would a person feel the need to repress positive ones? There are two reasons.

1. The abuser (prior to the event) may represent positives such as love, trust or companionship. Sexual abuse is such a violation of that love and trust that the abused may associate his pain with the previously experienced positive feelings. Since the violation of trust involves shifting feelings from good to bad, the abused may generalize from this experience to the belief that pleasure may ultimately lead to pain.

2. Such interpretations may lead to repression—the blocking of pleasure in order that pain will not follow. The result is the inability of the abused male to recognize and express pleasure in certain circumstances.

Pleasure may prove to be a threat as it relates to intimacy with significant others. Other areas of intimacy, however, which are perceived as less threatening, do not require unconscious protection.

The Case of John

John is a 40-year-old male who was sexually abused from the age of 12. John came to therapy to seek the answer to why he abruptly leaves situations just at the point where he might enjoy success and stability. This pattern of leaving has caused John to repeatedly "sell out and start over again." He is concerned that at age 40, he has accumulated little in assets and, although his janitorial business is becoming well established, he again has the urge to give it up.

John disclosed to me that he was sexually abused at the hands of certain authorities in a private school setting. He and other survivors have been part of a recent police investigation. John spoke of the abuse in some detail, but was reluctant (or unable) to describe feelings beyond ongoing anger.

John's wife joined therapy during the third session. She talked about John's need for control within the relationship and his frequent, spontaneous withdrawal from her for no apparent reason. She is very upset about the possibility of termination of the janitorial business and is threatening to leave the marriage.

John showed some comfort in discussing his patterns of behavior; however, he was disorganized and intense when the subject of feelings came up. As one would expect, his wife was at her limit of tolerance and insisted on discussing John's withdrawing from intimacy, his lack of love and affection, and his overall stoic nature. John's resistance to these discussions was so strong that I feared dropout from therapy. I even suggested that we stay with John's initial plan for therapy, which was to discuss behavior with a view toward change. But John failed to return for follow-up sessions and no progress was made. John's anxiety level was so high in the areas of love, trust and his success (an instance of pleasure) that he followed his old patterns of withdrawing under anxiety; that is, withdrawing from therapy.

We can learn much from John's case. Part of an abused male's defense system is the ability to repress feelings of pleasure when such feelings grow in intensity. High intensity of pleasure results in anxiety and the need for relief. Good feelings were automatically repressed to avoid the perceived ensuing pain, which for him follows pleasure. A tolerable distance was created through withdrawal. John's wife could not know that the intensity of his intimacy toward her was responsible for this withdrawal, which she thought originated in lack of love and affection.

John had the opportunity, through the years, to achieve success through his business ventures. His anxiety when approaching success may be attributed to fear of loss of that success; thus, we see repression at work again. The cycle of repression causes John to "sell out and move on" for self-protection. This drifting pattern results in a sense of meaninglessness, which John attempts to overcome by entering into a new venture. We are witnessing an emotionally exhausting and fruitless cycle in operation.

Whole and Partial Repression

A complication of repression can exist. Anna Freud stated that repression may be whole or partial. An abused male may feel pleasure at a mild or moderate level, but experience anxiety when pleasure grows to a strong level, as was the case with John. A mild or moderate level may include happiness, joy, being "turned on," etc. A strong level would include excitement, elation, euphoria. This is an example of partial repression. The anxiety is associated with emotions at an intense level but not a mild one. A different kind of partial repression is represented by the ability to recall a traumatic event in the past, but none of the feelings surrounding it.

The Case of Harry

Harry provides an example of whole, or total, repression. He had been referred to me by his therapist, who was at a loss to establish the reason for a "black emptiness" that Harry frequently referred to. Although Harry had made progress in some areas, the feeling of "black emptiness" was impairing exploration of symptoms of anger and distrust. After some preliminary work with Harry, it occurred to me that the significant others in his life, including his therapist, were treating this emptiness as an impairment and were trying to talk Harry into letting it go so further progress could be made. I decided to treat the unknown impairment as a feeling in itself and utilize a procedure called Visual Kinetic Disassociation, which encourages the client to re-experience old feelings associated with a traumatic event.

As Harry experienced the "black emptiness" during one session, I encouraged him to allow the emptiness to expand and to allow his mind to drift to the original situation in which he experienced this emptiness. Although he seemed to be blocked mentally at that point, I strongly encouraged him to pursue the feeling in spite of his obvious discomfort. Eventually, Harry expressed his dismay that there was nothing further to explore. There was simply a "black emptiness" that would not allow him to go any further. Obviously, something about the feeling was too terrible to relive. I refused to give up and Harry courageously continued to explore the emptiness. Our persistence was rewarded and he finally began to see through the darkness. This is what he said:

"The darkness is all around. I guess I'm about nine or ten years old. I see something. A spider. I'm in the attic and I'm hiding. My brother's friend is visiting again. He always manages to get me alone and make me do things to him [described later as oral and anal sex]. I hated what he made me do and I hated him. But he threatened me. I hid in the dark attic and barely breathed so he wouldn't find me. I imagined rats and spiders in the dark attic and was terrified. But I sat there rather than let him get me again. Nobody will ever know how I felt. I wished I would die and it would all go away."

Needless to say, the session was uncomfortable and filled with much emotion. In the end, we were able to address the trauma, and the client was eventually able to overcome the unknown "black emptiness." We were able to begin treatment on problem areas that were now clearer to us.

Repression of the attic scene served to save the child from perhaps going into a state of complete withdrawal. The resultant feelings of anger and mistrust persisted throughout the years without logical explanation. Harry required assistance to discover the cause of his dilemma.

This example illustrates total repression, which was the cause of the feeling of "black emptiness."

The Case of Bob

Another client, Bob, exemplifies partial repression. An adult male family friend took Bob (aged 13) to a part-time job experience with the blessing of the family. Halfway to the destination, the adult stopped the car and told the young man that he had something he wanted to show him. The "something" turned out to be several weapons. At first, the young man thought it was "cool," as he described it.

However, the weapons were used as a threat to control the youth while he was raped by the older person. Afterward, he was dropped off and told that he and his family would be killed if he ever told. When describing the incident, Bob, who was now in his mid-30s, was visibly upset, and no matter how hard he tried, he could not visualize the whole scene. Nor could he connect with his feelings during the rape, but he could describe his fear beforehand and confusion mixed with fear and anger afterward.

Bob exemplifies the ability to recall the whole of an abusive event. However, he has no recall of the emotions he experienced during the event. This is an example of the second kind of partial repression.

My work with abused males leads me to conclude that they are vulnerable to hurt, embarrassment, confusion and pleasure because of the act of abuse. All of these emotions may be partially affected in one individual, or just one or more may be affected while the others remain functional.

Not all defenses are maladaptive. Adaptive defenses, particularly those established at a mature phase, may protect the individual from anxiety while promoting healthy functioning. Repression in the abused male must fall into the category of maladaptive because it operates at the expense of healthy functioning. Its rapidity and pervasiveness can only lead to personality breakdown. The fact that sexually abused males survive at all under these circumstances is a tribute to their ingenuity and courage. They must use up enormous amounts of courage every day for simple tasks that others take for granted.

Steps to Recovery

Whether or not we explore past experiences or analyze the defenses that contribute to a person's emotional state, at some point the process of change through solution becomes the focus of therapy. Whether or not insight is of value in the direction of change depends on the person's viewpoint. One thing is certain:

change must be undertaken at some stage if positive growth is an expectation.

Before a person can make a move in the direction of recovery, a commitment must be made to reduce the energy expended on the past. The past cannot be changed and does not deserve much of our emotional energy. If sexually abused males are to overcome the effects of the abuse, recovery focus must be directed toward the here and now. Should a search through past experiences lead to a better understanding of repression and enhance development toward solution, we are obligated to carry out the search, but then we must return to the present and future.

Recent work of solution-focused therapists has produced excellent results by utilizing a person's ability to initiate his or her own solutions without a long-drawn-out focus on the past. I have witnessed sexually abused males change a dysfunctional behavior to a healthy behavior over a period of time, and this has resulted in weakened repression. This means that recovery can be approached at a behavioral level.

If sexual abuse of males is to be treated successfully, attention must be devoted to the three major symptoms that are common to male survivors—anger, mistrust and meaninglessness. These problem areas lead to immobilization of healthy functioning and poor decision-making ability. Recovery can result in self-fulfillment and success which may have been elusive throughout the years.

Chapter 2

Anger

Definition: "A feeling of great displeasure, hostility, indignation or exasperation."

Webster's Dictionary

Anger may be viewed in two different ways, or as two different types. One type of anger builds up inside until it has to be released. We may release our anger through various methods, such as physical activity, or allow it to build until it transfers to physical symptoms, such as headaches, tiredness or feelings of tension and unhappiness. Even at this level, symptoms may be relieved through expression of angry feelings.

A second type of anger is a reaction that can go out of control. This anger, which is triggered by annoyance or irritation, may lead to immediate violence. It is important to note that with this second type of anger, expression is not as appropriate as dissolving the anger before it gets out of control. A specialist in anger management may be called upon to assist the individual in learning ways of controlling this anger rather than expressing it.

The first type of anger, as a cause of symptoms, is a more common feature of sexually abused men than the second type, and a disturbing one. Within such men, anger is a constant—not usually displayed in spontaneous violence, but ever present beneath the surface of their emotions. It is responsible for the creation of ongoing conflict and unhappiness for the abused and significant others.

If we could go back to the original abusive event, we would see the abused male caught in the first type of anger, giving rise to a cycle of anger-producing symptoms.

1. The male child was seduced and sexually molested.

2. A series of emotions was produced—emotions such as hurt, guilt, confusion, fear and perhaps pleasure.

3. These emotions were not readily dealt with because of the immature state of the abused, and so they were repressed.

4. Inability to express or resolve the emotions led to frustration and anger.

5. Anger could not be expressed because of the threat of consequences.

6. Anger remained as an unconscious, learned response.

Anger becomes firmly established and continues in future interactions with others. Anger is ever present, but not in a spontaneous way—rather in a delayed, inappropriate way, and is expressed as need be, to whoever is handy, usually an unsuspecting significant other. The unsuspecting other, such as a caring spouse, a passive friend or the abused person's children, represent a safe target in a familiar environment. Since the abused male is caught in an unconscious cycle, he can neither understand nor control his behavior and experiences self-loathing for the actions he has directed at persons he loves.

In the case of a sexually abused male, ask a loved one if she recognizes the above process. I wager the answer would be "yes" in most instances. Since anger is constant and close to the surface, it may be expected that the trigger points would be reactions similar to the original emotions experienced during the abuse, which were later repressed. For example, when an abused male is confronted with situations giving rise to hurt, embarrassment, confusion or pleasure in the here and now, the response will be anger. To add to the complexity of the problem, anger may arise in a situation of intimacy or closeness to another. This would be especially true if the abused male had felt a closeness toward the abuser.

The Case of Mark

Mark, a mid-30s male survivor, exemplifies the inappropriate responses of anger resulting from repression. Mark's wife, during a joint session, described an incident that is typical of his behavior.

"Mark and I have had a couple of really good weeks. He seemed easygoing and stable. Last Friday night we had friends over and everyone was clowning around. The trouble started when Mark leaned back in his easy chair and tipped over. He went head-over-heels. We were all in a laughing mood anyway and this was really funny. Mark laughed too, but I guess I was the only one to notice that look which crossed his face. The look I have seen before—a danger signal of pending ugliness. Everyone continued to laugh and some comments were made about Mark, all in fun. I sensed Mark's withdrawal. When the last of our friends left, Mark flew into a rage. He screamed at me about my inconsideration and lack of caring about his feelings. As I tried to talk to him, he became more incensed and finally put me out of the house, locking the door. He continued to rant and rave until he was exhausted and went to the rec room after finally letting me back in. I had seen this behavior before, so I simply went to bed. In the morning, he apologized and looked like a sorry little kid."

Mark's wife is describing a cycle of repression/suppression, followed by inappropriate anger. Embarrassment, resulting from the chair incident, followed by (what Mark perceived as) hurtful comments reinforced Mark's feelings of insecurity. It was at that point that Mark repressed his feelings and became unable to deal with primary emotions such as embarrassment and hurt. Instead, anger proved to be his way out: an anger that is close to the surface at all times and displaced toward an innocent, safe other, namely, his wife. Mark confirmed that he felt terrible about the incident; his intense, inappropriate response was automatic. It resulted from an unconscious process over which he has no control. Mark and his wife could describe many such incidents, which reinforces that a pattern is in operation.

Mark displays a push/pull effect at the emotional level. His anger is near the surface and often displaced toward a loved one rather than expressed at the point of the initial cause. He is a tense man, often complaining of tiredness, muscular stiffness and headaches. His physician has given him a clean bill of health, which likely indicates the presence of psychosomatic problems.

The push/pull effect consists of a pull toward intimacy followed by an inappropriate push away from love and affection. Mark's wife describes sequences of closeness and then sudden, unexplained withdrawal. As an example, the couple spent a weekend, without the children, in a honeymoon-style setting. The couple indulged in sightseeing and candlelight dinners, and lovemaking. Upon return, Mark became quiet and withdrawn. He spent two nights sleeping on the couch while his wife cried herself to sleep. She stated that he seemed sullen and angry, and she avoided confrontation because she felt it would bring out his anger. Eventually, Mark followed his usual pattern of apologizing and his push toward intimacy.

Mark's experience of intense closeness proves too much for his emotional capabilities. He feels a need to distance himself in order to feel safe from vulnerability. After all, in Mark's unconscious, closeness would lead to hurt. Thus, emotional distance creates a sense of relief. These push/pull patterns are not exclusive to sexually abused males. They may show themselves in any case where a violation of trust has been experienced, especially in earlier life. However, it is a pattern worth looking for in sexually abused males who were violated by a known offender. Most offenders are known to their victims and are in a position of trust.

The Case of Ronald

We will do well to recognize repressed emotions and learn to deal with them. Anger is a likely alternative should we seek to avoid primary feelings.

In the sexually abused male, traumatic feelings are repressed at the point of impact in the original abusive event; however, the process of repression establishes these feelings as an ongoing force in the here and now. The only *conscious* feeling is anger.

A case in point is Ronald, a man who was sexually abused in a training school 30 years ago. Ronald had progressed in therapy and was at the point where he felt a need to explore his past in order to gain further understanding of his present feelings and behaviors. Let's examine a transcript from one of our sessions, where he exemplified repression in its truest form.

Ronald: "Everyone was getting ready for bed and I stood before him. He had called me into his office for some reason. I figured I must have done something wrong and was about to be punished. He told me to take off my underwear. He stood behind me. Then, I felt his thing rubbing between my legs and he kept saying how beautiful I was. Then he came all over me. I got cleaned off and dressed. He then said I could leave. He also told me that this was a secret. If I kept being a good boy, I would soon be his favorite and get extra rewards."

Therapist: "Are you okay to go on?"

Ronald: "Well . . . that's about it, what happened."

Therapist: "You wanted to talk about feelings. Can I ask you how you felt at the time this was happening?"

Ronald: "Well . . . sure, I'm pissed off, just talking about it."

Therapist: "Ron, I'm not sure I understand. You are pissed off now, but how did you feel then?"

Ronald: *"How would you feel if some dirty old son-of-a-bitch put his thing all over you? Just try to think how you would feel."*

Therapist: *"I can't imagine. You seem very angry now."*

Ronald: *"Sure, I'm angry. The whole thing is sick."*

Therapist: *"Well, at least you can tell me your feelings today."*

Ronald: *"Couldn't you see ...I'm embarrassed. I'm ashamed of myself for standing there while he was doing that to me. I really wish he had beaten me instead. I always thought he was the one who would someday tell my parents that I was fine and could go home."*

When we see evidence of repression, we would do well to pay close attention to the language of the client. Ronald speaks of feelings in the here and now, but is not able to describe *past* embarrassment, fear and shame as he continues the conversation with the therapist. However, the feelings evoked during the conversation mirror the feelings that were evoked during the abuse. This is reinforced by the fact that Ronald quickly turns to anger when he is confronted by these emotions in the present situation, just as he is known to do in his daily life. He is able to deal effectively with certain other negative emotions, but not these three.

Perhaps the best way to demonstrate the phenomenon of anger is the Iceberg Theory. An iceberg presents one-ninth of its force on the surface. Eight-ninths remain hidden to the viewer, under the surface. Anger and the hidden primary feelings have an iceberg effect, as shown in Illustration 1.

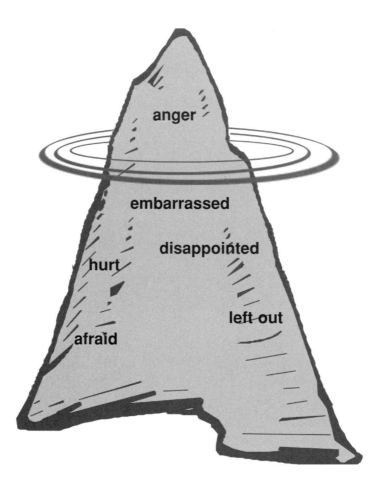

ILLUSTRATION 1

Often we cannot perceive the underlying forces. Whenever I make this analogy with a client, I cannot help but think of the *Titanic*. I often show the illustration to a client and tell him that, as captain of his own ship, he can avoid disaster by learning to pay attention to underlying forces and deal with them.

Most sexually abused men I have met have been in a state of constant anger. They are masters at suppressing their anger. This anger distorts listening skills, common-sense judgment, sense of humor and perception of others' intentions. Moreover, if we were to review the life of these men, it would become apparent that anger has caused immense damage to relationships.

Anger Recovery

First and foremost, anger must be translated to a primary feeling (such as hurt, guilt, embarrassment, fear, etc.). I have met few sexually abused men who have a basic knowledge of their emotional system. For example, one man described sadness over not being with his children after separating from his wife. Treatment was not effective initially, until it occurred to me that he was not in a state of sadness; rather, he was feeling guilty.

Certainly the treatment issues differ. Another client was concerned about what he felt was an anxiety disorder. After some discussion, I learned that this anxiety surfaced during frequent interviews with management figures at the workplace. Our eventual conclusion was that this was indeed appropriate nervousness under the circumstances. There was no anxiety disorder.

To translate anger to primary feelings requires a great deal of "new" thinking. Sexually abused men, rather than avoiding certain feelings as society has conditioned them to do, need to become fully aware of all of their feelings. Furthermore, in itself, translating anger into primary feelings will not lead to recovery. But it will constitute the first step. The following three-step approach to recovery has been very helpful to sexually abused men.

Step 1

Step 1 consists of a conscious, deliberate attempt to block anger. Anger is an opportunity to recognize and acknowledge primary feelings. Because of the nature of anger, an abused man may miss that opportunity, if he allows anger to proceed beyond what is clearly the first signal. The first signal may take the form of butterflies in the stomach, a feeling of blushing, or shakiness, to name a few. Recognizing the first signal does not usually pose a problem. It is at this stage, the initial signal, that anger must be suppressed in any way a person knows how. Whether he bites his tongue, pinches himself or holds his breath, the purpose will be served if he blocks any further anger. This kind of suppression of anger, on its own, can be harmful; thus we move to step 2.

Step 2

A search for and recognition of the primary feeling should be completed during the second step. This may be a very difficult process for a man who has used anger and other methods to avoid certain emotions. This difficulty may be overcome, however, by learning more about emotions and how they fall into levels of intensity. Illustration 2 is a table with helpful listings of feelings. A search through the table can help to determine the most accurate word(s) to describe what feeling came before the anger. The man should try to recall a recent angry moment and work backward to recall details of the incident, in order to determine what feeling may have preceded the anger. He simply picks out from the table the word that comes to mind as he recalls the event. A significant other, or therapist, may be helpful in completing the process with him. Let us say a co-worker may have called him an uncomplimentary name and he became angry. He may have initially felt hurt, or disrespected, or inadequate, before shifting to anger. In some cases there may be difficulty because masters of avoiding emotions can move to anger so quickly. In these cases he must persevere with the process, because a primary emotion *always* precedes the anger.

Particular attention must be given to step 2. Repression limits the knowledge of our feelings and leaves us with a narrow spectrum of emotions. A man must not attempt to express within his limited spectrum, but instead must use the lists in the table in order to advance his knowledge of the whole emotional system. Getting stuck would lead to discouragement; therefore, he must take the time for further education in the area of feelings.

Step 3

Completion of step 3 involves expression of the primary feeling. A solution-focused approach, based on the philosophy that the person with the problem has the capacity to solve the problem, is paramount. How the emotion is expressed is a personal choice, since an expression used by one person may not work for another. Many of my clients have explored different choices of personal expressions until the most comfortable was found. It is imperative that others avoid telling a person how to express; for example, encouraging a man to cry if he is sad assumes that the crying would be helpful. But crying, for some people, is not a positive response. The following strategies for expression of feelings were developed by three different clients, as responses to negative comments.

1. "As I searched for my expression, I couldn't help but think of my grandfather, who only hears what he wants to. I became enamored of selective hearing. I simply choose not to hear the comment and go about my business. It really works for me."

Vocabulary of Feelings: Anger

	Depressed	Inadequate	Fearful
STRONG	desolate depressed hopeless alienated gloomy dismal bleak in despair empty barren grieved grief grim	worthless good for nothing washed up powerless helpless impotent crippled inferior emasculated useless finished like a failure	terrified frightened intimidated horrified desperate panicky terror stricken stage fright dread vulnerable paralyzed
MODERATE	distressed upset downcast sorrowful demoralized discouraged miserable pessimistic tearful weepy rotten awful horrible terrible blue lost melancholy	inadequate whipped defeated incompetent inept overwhelmed ineffective lacking deficient unable incapable small insignificant like Casper milquetoast unfit unimportant incomplete no good immobilized	afraid scared fearful apprehensive jumpy shaky threatened distrustful risky alarmed butterflies awkward defensive
MILD	unhappy down low bad blah disappointed sad glum	lacking confidence unsure of yourself uncertain weak inefficient	nervous anxious unsure hesitant timid shy worried uneasy on edge embarrassed ill at ease doubtful

ILLUSTRATION 2

Confused	Hurt	Lonely	Guilt/Shame
bewildered puzzled battled perplexed trapped confounded in a dilemma befuddled in a quandary full of questions confused	crushed destroyed ruined degraded pain(ed) wounded devastated tortured disgraced humiliated anguished at the mercy of cast off forgotten rejected discarded	isolated abandoned all alone forsaken cut off	sick at heart unforgivable humiliated disgraced degraded horrible mortified exposed
mixed up disorganized foggy troubled adrift lost at loose ends going around in circles disconcerted frustrated in a bind ambivalent disturbed helpless embroiled	hurt belittled shot down overlooked abused depressed criticized detained censured discredited disparaged laughed at maligned mistreated ridiculed devalued scorned mocked scoffed at used debased slammed impugned exploited cheapened slandered	lonely alienated estranged remote alone apart from others isolated from others	ashamed guilty remorseful crummy to blame lost face demeaned
uncertain unsure bothered uncomfortable undecided	put down neglected overlooked minimized let down unappreciated taken for granted	left out excluded lonesome distant aloof	regretful wrong embarrassed at fault in error responsible for blew it goofed lament

2. "I like the concept of power and control. I now view disturbing comments as an invitation to respond intensely, but I don't accept the invitation. I say to myself, 'Not this time, thank you. I want to keep power over my emotions instead of turning them over to you. These emotions are mine, not yours, and I'll do what I want with them.'"

3. "I'm amazed at the response of people when I express my feelings. I might say, 'You are entitled to your opinion, but I don't have to agree.' I can now remain cool and calm. How they react to that is for them to work out. I never knew this could be so easy. My anger is all but non-existent these days."

Great responses! Instead of allowing harmful primary feelings to build up through shifting to anger, expression allows immediate resolution of these feelings. Once men experience this kind of success, nothing can stop their progress.

The three-step approach to recovering from anger has proven successful for men who commit to it. This is not a magical solution. It should be approached as hard work that requires practice. Immediate recovery is virtually impossible, but practice and perseverance will result in gradual progress and permanent success. Small successes accumulate over time, and a person should recognize and celebrate each and every success. Learning elimination of anger can be viewed in the same way as learning to play the piano: one doesn't learn to do it without discipline and practice. But someday, what is awkward and difficult now will feel natural and comfortable.

Chapter 3
Mistrust

Definition: "To lack confidence in; to doubt or suspect."
Webster's Dictionary

The extent to which we carry confidence in others into adulthood depends on experiences during earlier developmental stages when we were vulnerable, both physically and emotionally. It is during these stages that we begin the process of judging the behavior and intent of others.

The majority of sexually abused men utilize defense systems that reflect their learned inability to achieve confidence in others, because of earlier negative experiences. People ask me why they should trust their spouses, friends, co-workers, etc. They usually respond with surprise when I state that perhaps learning to trust or distrust is not a significant issue. In fact, trust should not be an issue in any relationship; abused men should not struggle to restore their ability to trust others.

Further explanation is needed about why trust should not be an issue. At birth we are subject to the "luck of the draw." Should our luck provide us with caring and protective parents, we are likely to mature in a non-threatening environment, which results in a natural state of confidence in our ability to cope with everyday interactions. Trust is not an issue of concern. Mistrust, on the other hand, may be learned should significant others fail to provide care and encouragement and to create a safe environment.

Imagine the learned mistrust of a person who is subjected to abuse (usually ongoing) during a vulnerable early stage of development and is not rescued. Such an extreme of mistrust may be incomprehensible to many of us. The sexually abused male experiences extreme pain and suffering resulting from the violation of his mind and body, leading to a high level of mistrust.

Men who are in need of a resolution of the pain of violation often try to fill this need by generalizing mistrust. They adopt the strategy of a general distrust of others, minimum self-disclosure and masking of feelings in order to avoid further pain at the hands of others. It stands to reason that such strategies lead to broken relationships and lack of positive sense of self throughout their adult years.

Behind such strategies lie fear—fear concerning the intent of others based on previous experiences of trust violation. Arthur Jersild best described the phenomenon of generalization of fear. He stated that the essential element when such a spread of fear takes place is the fact that something left the person in a state of apprehension about fear, or fear of fear. This conditioning process does not in itself create a new fear, but provides an object or circumstance with which his fright becomes associated.

Sexually abused men often fail to disclose their fears. Jersild states that by virtue of the premium that is placed on not being afraid, or revealing that he is afraid, a child may be driven to the point that one of his fears is simply that of showing fear.

Jersild is describing the mechanics of the very basis of mistrust. The object that creates conditioning of fright in sexually abused men is the significant other, often a trusted person. Such fear may manifest itself as mistrust of others in general and escalate as the abused encounters closeness or intimacy. It is conceivable that the more significant the other becomes, the more mistrust is experienced. As you may recall, such phenomena do not necessarily occur at the conscious level. A stranger may elicit an automatic mistrust; an authority figure, more mistrust; a loved one, even more extreme mistrust. The degree of fear or mistrust can be correlated with the significance of the other.

The fear of showing fear becomes an important factor in the abused male's behavior. Rather than show fear and become vulnerable, the adult male goes through a series of unhealthy behaviors that create distance from others, thus relieving the vulnerability that closeness elicits. Once distance is achieved, the man may begin to move closer again. Significant others may describe this as a push/pull effect, based on mistrust of intimacy.

Repression explains the push/pull effect. Repressed feelings of fear, hurt, shame and confusion are reawakened from the unconscious when the abused encounters intimacy at a sufficient level to create vulnerability. Sadly, love becomes one such trigger. As one of my clients stated, "You can't hurt me if you're not important to me."

Repressed feelings are not resolved feelings, but instead sit in the unconscious waiting to reawaken when an object similar to the original object comes along. Defenses such as repression become stronger and more rigid with maturity; therefore, if a man hopes to outgrow his automatic responses such as mistrust, he may find himself waiting a whole lifetime.

The Case of Bill

In 1992 I met Bill, a 37-year-old married man who was sexually abused during childhood. He is a sensitive, caring man who is a good provider and loves his wife and family.

Bill was referred to me by his therapist of two years. She was concerned about lack of recent progress in overcoming what Bill described as his black mood. Symptoms of the black mood included overwhelming dread followed by numbing of feelings. This led to a withdrawal from others as Bill became quiet and preferred to go off alone and avoid contact with anyone. Bill's relationship with his family and co-workers had suffered over the years and he described his life as "going through the motions" during the frequent black mood periods. He was feeling discouraged and guilty over his behavior, particularly since he and others were unable to explain the pattern. He had gained the reputation of being cold and moody.

Bill's problems were twofold. One, he was unaware of his protective mechanisms, which created his responses and subsequent behavior. Two, he was unable to express his fears to others, as he would become more vulnerable.

Through our discussions, Bill was able to understand the unconscious drives that caused his behavior and undertook with me the difficult task of behaving differently from the way he felt when experiencing his learned responses. On one occasion, Bill and his wife enjoyed a night out without the children. They both experienced closeness as they dined and danced throughout the evening. The following day, Bill felt his black mood coming on. This was his usual signal to withdraw from closeness. Instead of acting upon his black mood, he stopped off at a florist's and bought his wife flowers with a note saying, "I love you. Thanks for a wonderful evening." Bill reported that his new behavior brought about a warm feeling, which replaced the black mood.

My job as a therapist was to encourage Bill to behave in a manner that was the direct opposite of his learned responses. He needed the experience of expressing closeness, as difficult as that might be. Bill experienced first-hand that his gentle behavior did not bring on rejection, as his mistrust had led him to expect; instead, his wife was surprised and delighted. The courage required for Bill to undertake this simple act of affection cannot be emphasized enough, in light of the power of learned, automatic mistrust responses. It was important that Bill take a risk and learn that he would be okay. Bill has since replaced his philosophy of "You can't hurt me if you're not important to me" with "There is less chance of you hurting me if I show you I love you." Bill learned to accept a fact of life. There are no guarantees that we will not be hurt by others. However, there is no need to bring about the very hurt we wish to avoid by pushing others away.

It is imperative that men begin to learn that they can cope with unacceptable behavior of others because they are not now the helpless children they were when they were abused. Bill and I spent several sessions discussing his new-found freedom and new ways to maintain his healthy behavior. His success may be partly explained by his receptiveness to learning new questions in order to seek new answers. For example, when he encountered a negative feeling, Bill learned to ask, "How can I move away from this feeling?" This question replaces his old question, "Why am I feeling this way?" Bill developed a list of new, action questions that would lead to positive outcomes.

Although everyone who tried to reason with Bill over the years told him he had to learn to be more trusting, Bill and I did not spend time on that subject. He focused on becoming the nice person he really is and developed a strong appreciation for his own strengths. He seldom thinks of trust now, for his trust is within himself.

As a therapist, I have come to terms with the fact that mistrust will manifest itself in many ways as a sexually abused man interacts with others. I take such manifestations as a signal to elicit ways in which to boost self-esteem rather than try to convince the man that trust is a good thing and he is hurting others by his behavior. Such an approach would surely drive the man away from therapy. If we view mistrust as an opportunity to develop faith in oneself, we may never need to convince men such as Bill that trust is appropriate. Trust and mistrust are learned responses. A person need never think of the consequences of either if he has faith in his own being and his ability to cope.

Recovery from Mistrust

I have never met a self-actualized man who was concerned about trust. Self-actualization means that a person fulfills his own needs and is not overly concerned about the opinions of others. Whether or not a man is concerned about what others think is a learned response. Men who were sexually abused as children have already lost self-focus and exaggerate the importance of what others think.

The Case of Michael

As an example of potential losses and fear, I would like to introduce you to Michael, one of my former clients. He had been contemplating disclosure of his sexual abuse to his best friend, who happened to be his brother-in-law. Michael felt that disclosure would help him resolve his issues and give him a support network beginning with his friend. Upon disclosure, Michael was met with silence. He was very hurt. His brother-in-law avoided any conversation around the disclosure and changed the subject. Michael was further dismayed when his brother-in-law began to avoid contact with him, and the friendship soon dissolved. Michael's mistrust became more rigid following this event and he became more closed than ever.

Michael, like other sexually abused men, needs to develop confidence in himself and stop being concerned about what others think. Even though rejection may have been experienced, Michael will benefit by learning that he can live through it. In fact, if he can develop a strong sense of self-worth, his confidence will be restored and mistrust will no longer be an issue.

The most effective way for Michael to develop confidence is through a gradual movement toward feeling safe and secure within himself. Instead of dwelling on why he became mistrustful, Michael and I concentrated on answering the question, "How are you going to move away from mistrust and toward feeling secure?" By security here we really mean self-value, which can be achieved through investing in oneself. This concept was difficult for Michael to internalize, and required a step-by-step approach in order to minimize the pain of changing lifelong patterns of behavior.

Michael's story represents a successful outcome, which can be achieved by anyone who decides to commit to such change. The following model, which Michael and I used, established the necessary framework for gradual change and provides a measure for progress. Also, the solutions are Michael's and not those imposed by the therapist. I consider these factors vital to success.

We commenced the process of change by using a scale to measure Michael's present state of self-value and then his desired state. This model was taken from the works of I. Berg's solution-focused therapy. Let's review the process as it worked for Michael.

SELF-VALUE

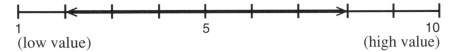

1   5   10
(low value)   (high value)

Michael determined that he was presently scoring 2 on the scale and stated that this figure was probably indicative of his lifetime score. He also determined that he would like to work up to 8 and maintain that level as a lifelong goal. One of the major reasons for failure to change is that people try to change all at once and are unable to maintain such large changes. In other words, they try to change from 2 to 8. Now we see the importance of the scale, for gradual change increases the potential for success.

Michael's goals were set after some discussion to ensure they were appropriate for the score on the scale. Likely smaller change will be appropriate at the beginning and larger change toward the end. A review of Michael's achieved goals will illustrate how he advanced.

SCORE	ACHIEVED GOAL
2 → 3	Made a list of strengths that may have been displayed through the week.
3 → 4	Provided himself with small treats at least three times during the week.
4 → 5	Decided to say no to a request that he considered to be an imposition. This would be a change from the norm for him.
5 → 6	Acted in accordance with what he felt was to his own good without worrying about the opinions of others. This goal would continue for a three-week period, after which the results would be discussed during a session.
6 → 7	Spent two weeks with a focus on control over his own emotions. This meant that Michael would determine how he wanted to feel and would disregard negative, learned responses.

Michael's success can be attributed to several factors:

1. Michael was determined, and disregarded small failures as he sought to accomplish his goals.

2. Goals (which really represent solutions) were *elicited* by the therapist and were not suggested or imposed.

3. Michael was encouraged to determine the amount of time he needed between sessions to complete the goals. This

ensured that he advanced at his own pace rather than the pace I might incorrectly determine for him.

4. Michael was warned about the difficulty of the process he was about to undertake. I wanted no surprises in this regard.

Courage was an important factor in this process, and Michael persevered magnificently through the completion of the whole endeavor.

One question that is sometimes asked about this method of recovery is whether the person might not develop narcissism, or an excessive love for himself. But I would not be concerned about this issue, considering the extreme lack of self-focus sexually abused men exhibit.

Michael's wife joined us in one of our final sessions and confirmed his progress. She was excited and pleased about his progress and his ability to maintain it. She commented to me, "This is the man I knew he could be. After all these years, what happened?" As I was pondering my response about the clinical process, Michael answered, "I just do things differently these days." I found that there was nothing I could add. This was a simple but profound description of the whole outcome.

Michael continued to seek new ways in which to enrich his life, and his family and friends received the benefit of his new outlook. Several years later he had not looked back, and symptoms were not recurring. When I asked Michael about his problem with mistrust, he informed me that he didn't think about it these days.

This treatment approach may seem simplistic, but the treatment does not have to be complex. This is not to say that Michael and I did not discuss certain issues that caused resistance as he proceeded through the various steps. In this particular case, Michael and I worked hard to resolve his sense of guilt, which arose when he began focusing on himself instead of others. Such issues will emerge as progress is undertaken, and this indicates that a support system, such as a therapist, adds to the possibility of full recovery.

This is as complex as it gets. To eliminate mistrust, invest in your own happiness and success, without guilt, and mistrust will not be an issue. The object of mistrust is not the other person; rather, it is lack of confidence in coping with a potential loss. Develop faith in yourself and learn more about your strengths and coping skills. Learn to love yourself and the ability to love others will follow.

Chapter 4

Meaninglessness

Definition: "Having no significance or meaning; senseless."
Funk & Wagnall's Standard Dictionary

Meaning refers to sense or coherence; in its broadest sense, it is not to be confused with purpose, which constitutes putting forward an intention. In discussions of meaning, one may inquire into cosmic meaning—the coherent pattern or ordering of the universe (the meaning of life). One may also inquire into terrestrial meaning—goal or goals to which one applies oneself (the meaning of *my* life). Terrestrial meaning embraces purpose. A person who possesses a sense of meaning experiences life as having a purpose or function to be fulfilled, goals to be achieved. To live without meaning (meaninglessness) provokes considerable distress.

In this chapter, we shall look at how a sexually abused man proceeds to construct meaning. I have witnessed in male survivors, in the therapeutic setting, evidence of a tension between their human aspiration and their indifference. This indifference is what I refer to as meaninglessness.

The Case of Gordon

As I was thinking about this important chapter, a young woman approached me and asked if I would see her fiancé, Gordon. She described Gordon as a promising young man whom she loved dearly. Her concern lay in the fact that he moved from job to job frequently without a solid base for doing so. In fact, when he was on the verge of promotion, he would get restless and talk about resigning. He carried out that threat several times and went to work for another company. His fiancée felt a need to address this issue before marriage. She was confused by Gordon's patterns and concerned about their future as a couple under such unstable circumstances. Many discussions between the two had led her to believe that Gordon had no more understanding of his behavior than she had.

I met with Gordon shortly thereafter. He was a willing talker and promptly informed me that he had experienced the therapeutic setting in the past; in fact, he had been through several types of programs over a six-year period. He disclosed that he had been sexually active with older sisters as a child and was tormented for years by negative feelings and behavior. These feelings prompted him to participate in programs that were targeted toward recovery. I was not surprised to learn that he had invested a great deal in recovering from ongoing anger and resentment toward others, which had been resolved through previous therapy. The resentment he had felt could be described as mistrust, and Gordon was in agreement with that interpretation. It seemed to me that Gordon had overcome two of the three problems described in this book. At least anger and mistrust were more manageable at this point in his life than they had been at any other.

Gordon implied that happiness and fulfillment had eluded him over the years. He stated that he enjoys success but soon becomes indifferent to his progress and has difficulty giving sufficient effort for further accomplishment. He desired something meaningful and long-lasting, something that would provide a sense of achievement. As the interview progressed, Gordon disclosed that he was fearful of meaninglessness finding its way into his future marriage. His bride-to-be was unaware that he was considering breaking the engagement rather than taking the risk of a marriage commitment.

Later in the chapter I shall describe how Gordon recovered from his sense of meaninglessness. I would like to note first that the dissolution of meaning, the eroding of the foundations on which life rests, must be understood as a common clinical syndrome that is not exclusive to sexually abused men. However, I have had to explore this syndrome in every case where I treated male survivors.

C. G. Jung wrote, "Absence of meaning in life plays a crucial role in the aetiology of neurosis. A neurosis must be understood, ultimately, as a suffering of the soul which has not discovered its meaning . . . about a third of my cases are not suffering from any clinically definable neurosis but from the senselessness and aimlessness of their lives."

The problem of meaning in life is a significant one. Therapists must confront it frequently in everyday clinical work. The question of meaning is perplexing, and often people attempt to transform it into some lesser but more manageable question. I believe that the sexually abused man in particular must not shrink from the challenge of meaning, but must develop growth toward establishing a meaning that only he can fulfill.

Victor Frankl states that unique meanings fall into three categories:

1. what one accomplishes or gives to the world in terms of creations;

2. what one takes from the world in terms of encounters and experiences;

3. one's stand toward suffering, toward the fate that one cannot change.

"What matters," Frankl says, "is not how large is the radius of your activities but how well you fill the circle."

How well you fill its circle may actually mean engaging life to its fullest rather than plunging into the problems of meaninglessness. The question of meaning in life is, as the Buddha taught, not edifying. One must immerse oneself in the river of life and let the question of meaning drift away.

One of my dilemmas as a therapist has been the question of how to help a client immerse himself in the river of life. The question is particularly difficult when dealing with unmotivated clients who suffer from depression or learned helplessness. In the case of sexually abused men, repressed feelings may impair their ability to move forward toward risk-taking, which would enhance immersion in life's experiences.

As I searched for a strategy to assist clients with this problem, I kept in mind the fact that immersing oneself in life is the answer and did not attempt to directly approach the question of meaning. I believe that I may have solved the riddle through a model that focuses on balance, the one clue nature gave us toward peace and contentment.

Recovery from Meaninglessness

How does a person immerse himself in life and feel contentment? Let's examine three general areas of functioning in which most people operate. The following, I believe, represents the ideal balance.

AREAS OF FUNCTIONING

WORK
    (includes anything we consider work)   33.3%
PERSONAL RELATIONSHIPS
    (with anyone who is important to us)   33.3%
PERSONAL FOCUS
    (anything we do for our physical
    or emotional well-being)   33.3%

The theory behind balancing is simple. The more balance, the more contentment. The more imbalance, the more distress. Crisis throws us out of balance and, as we recover, we strive to gain balance. However, at any time we may adopt a lifestyle that represents imbalance and experience ongoing distress. It is not necessarily the case that material wealth fosters balance. For example, some very wealthy persons experience much distress because of imbalance, while some disadvantaged persons are able to lead a life of contentment because they have been able to create balanced functioning.

If we can shift our areas of functioning into balance we will be able to avoid much of the distress of everyday living and achieve meaning by engaging in all areas. This model can be used in the therapeutic setting or by any individual to assess and monitor the degree of balance in his or her life.

During my therapy with sexually abused men, it became apparent that care has to be taken in defining the meaning of each area of functioning in order that a person can accurately evaluate their present percentages. Of ultimate importance is the fact that the percentages represent emotional energy expended in that area of functioning. For example, should you spend one hour at your workplace daydreaming about your new car, that hour must be credited to personal focus and not work.

Definitions

WORK

This area represents anything that we consider work. It will certainly have different meanings for different people. For instance, a man who works in an office may look forward to mowing his lawn, while a man with a physical job may dread the same chore. The physical activity is the same, but the emotional attitudes toward the activity differ.

A problem exists in the overlapping of the three areas of functioning. This is evident in the case where a person enjoys the work he does. Would this not represent personal focus? Absolutely not. Work is work, whether we enjoy it or not. I know this may sound contradictory, and many workaholics justify the imbalance by stating they enjoy their work. They also die young because of heart failure, ulcers or other stress-related illnesses.

Should your work prove satisfying, it is not out of line to shift a small percentage to personal focus, but only a small portion. Activities outside the workplace must be evaluated on the spirit in which we approach them, such as the lawn-mowing chore. Another good example is the health club. If we dread our workout, it is probably work. If we revel in the sweat and strain, it represents personal focus.

PERSONAL RELATIONSHIPS

This is an area in which many people may come up with an inaccurate evaluation. One of my clients assessed his personal relationship with his wife at 5% because the couple had been in constant conflict and he was usually very angry about the relationship. Upon further consideration, he concluded that the relationship was a constant cause of pain and anger, and therefore represented as much as 70% of his emotional expenditure.

The point is that energy expended may be negative as well as positive. To evaluate this area of functioning, we must consider persons who are important to us; so again we see that the areas of functioning are personal and specific to each individual. For example, one person may place great emphasis on interactions with co-workers, while another person may find this same group of people of little importance.

The key to good assessment is to consider everyone who may be important to you and evaluate how much time you spend physically and mentally interacting with these significant others. You may have guessed by now that persons who are distrustful, angry or intense about others in some other way may display a high percentage in this area. On the other hand, persons who are self-determined may show a proportion closer to a balanced 33.3%.

PERSONAL FOCUS

Anything we do for our physical and emotional well-being would fall into this category. Care must be taken in our evaluation because there is an overlap with other areas. Enjoyable, independent activities such as reading, painting, craft-making, etc. are easy to evaluate. But suppose we go for a long walk in the park with the children; are we to evaluate such an activity as work, personal relationships or focus? Certainly there is an overlap; however, if you find this activity very enjoyable you experience well-being and should place your walk in the area of personal focus. If your interaction with the children is stronger, then personal relationship is the correct category. If you carry out this activity in a babysitting role, then it is work. A college course taken to promote one's position of employment is considered work. Should we take the course for our own enjoyment, then we are concerned with our personal focus. While the overlap exists, simply asking ourselves the intent of what we are doing or the spirit in which we are doing it will result in the most accurate evaluation.

Earlier in the chapter I introduced Gordon, a young man who was discontented and felt stuck in his unhappiness. Gordon and I completed an evaluation of his personal functioning and came up with the following:

WORK	70%
PERSONAL RELATIONSHIPS	25%
PERSONAL FOCUS	5%

Gordon was constantly throwing his energy into his work. With such a high work-related focus, it was perhaps impossible to set realistic expectations and goals around his job performance. Work was simply too important to him, and this had the result of exaggerating its importance and distorting his judgment in work-related matters. Also significant was his very low sense of self-importance, which was evident in the 5% personal focus. Gordon's absence of investment in his own well-being was indicative of a low sense of self-importance, and indeed may have been the result of it. Gordon usually felt selfish or guilty when he concentrated on his own happiness.

Gordon's personal relationships deserve examination. He was very much aware of his image with co-workers and put about 20% of his emotional energy into that function. This left 5% for his fiancée and others, a figure that was indicative of his withdrawal from them. Little wonder Gordon was having second thoughts about marriage.

Consideration must be given to the fact that Gordon did not have full awareness of his patterns nor of what force motivated his actions. Nor was he able to share his deepest thoughts and concerns with his fiancée. Thus, we have two young people who were afraid and confused.

When undertaking movement toward recovery, we must follow a very important rule. Go to the weak area and strengthen it instead of trying to reduce the strong area. You will find such a rule makes establishing recovery goals simpler and more realistic.

During Gordon's therapy, we targeted personal focus as the area for goal-work. After some deliberation, Gordon decided to commit himself to the following: (1) take daily early-morning walks, (2) build model cars, and (3) join a dart club. All three goals represented activities Gordon had once enjoyed, at different times in his life. Obviously, it would have been impossible for the therapist to set such meaningful goals on Gordon's behalf.

Within one month Gordon reported an improvement in his overall functioning. The energy he had recently devoted to personal focus led to a reduction in his work focus, as he left work earlier to participate in personal activities. Further goals were then established with regard to creating enjoyable activities with his fiancée, such as going out to dinner once a week and taking hikes in the country with her on Sundays.

Gordon experienced some resistance to these changes periodically and required encouragement to continue with his goal-work. As he persisted in his efforts, the resistance diminished. A re-evaluation of his personal functioning later on in the therapy showed the following results:

WORK	45%
PERSONAL RELATIONSHIPS	30%
PERSONAL FOCUS	25%

As a result of the shift in his personal functioning, he reported that his employer was expressing positive comments about his recent performance and he was deriving more satisfaction from his relationships. His increase in personal focus resulted in a better sense of his own importance as he invested in his well-being. The couple began to feel more confident, and during one of our last sessions his fiancée confirmed that she saw a remarkable change in Gordon. They eventually married and at last report were doing well together.

There have been other cases where I have seen results similar to those achieved by Gordon. Commitment to goals and the courage to persevere when resistance is present are the necessary ingredients for success. Achieving the best possible balance results in restoration of emotional stability. Since goal-work produces more activities, a person becomes busier with tasks of their own choosing—busy enough to be immersing themselves in life.

Some people instinctively balance their lives; others are taught how to do so through the family system or other significant sources. For the sexually abused male, I hope he will trust the theory and guidelines in this chapter to improve the quality of his life and discover meaning in doing so.

Chapter 5

The Therapeutic Process

Dynamics of the Client– Therapist Relationship

All sexually abused men require counseling. Although it is widely accepted that female abuse survivors require counseling, it is less well recognized that males do.

The male abuse survivor going into counseling should understand the dynamics of the client–therapist relationship. This will enable him to know what to expect and will result in more effective treatment.

Preceding chapters describe how anger, mistrust and meaninglessness impair healthy functioning of survivors, potentially for a lifetime. The dynamics of the client–therapist relationship may play out a similar script, in which the three major symptoms impair the development of a warm and trusting relationship, which is necessary to facilitate change. The sexually abused male will likely act out the three symptoms in therapy, usually early in the process.

Anger may manifest itself early in therapy in the form of harsh criticism of others, or even of therapists in general for not having provided solutions in past therapy. The tone would be such that the therapist might be tempted to intervene with an attempt to soften the conversation. Mistrust is a given characteristic of the male survivor and will be in evidence as he questions the competence of the therapist, the ability of the therapist to care sincerely or issues related to confidentiality. Meaninglessness is a frustrating quality to bring to therapy, as it may show up in the inability to set therapeutic goals and proceed toward solutions. These problems occur when the abused questions the value of therapy and the possibility of a positive outcome.

When the symptoms under discussion are present, the therapeutic process may be threatened very early by premature termination. The creation of an open and trusting relationship will not be an easy process because of the previous negative life experiences of the survivor. It would stand to reason that the abused male would test the safety of the setting and, just as important, would experience automatic or unconscious negative responses to defend against the warmth and intimacy of the therapist's approach.

Both the therapist and the survivor have certain responsibilities during the early stages. Abuse survivors have the responsibility to view therapy as what it really is: a unique relationship unlike any other they have experienced to date. Their role is to participate with a view to achieving the desired outcome. The therapist has a responsibility to provide a warm and emotionally safe environment and to persevere through the acting-out of major symptoms, especially anger. This may not be an easy feat so early in the setting.

I have found it helpful in my practice to periodically review the social work values and principles set out by Felix Biestek in *The Casework Relationship.* Not only do Biestek's principles help me to persevere through difficult times in therapy; they also represent, to a considerable degree, an environment that is foreign to the survivor in its unconditional acceptance. I believe it is worthwhile to outline the principles here and incorporate them into the therapy.

Individualization. Every individual, group or community is unique and deserving of consideration. Each individual has dignity and worth, on his or her own merit.

Purposeful expression of feeling. Every individual has the need to express feelings. Their right to do so is basic to social work. Emotions are as important as thoughts or beliefs or knowledge, and negative emotions are as important as positive emotions.

Controlled emotional environment. Every individual has a right to expect that someone will be able to relate to his level of feeling. A worker must be able to feel with another, not just talk with him. The worker need not have the same feelings, but he or she must show understanding of the feelings of another person.

Acceptance. Every individual has a right to be accepted for what he is, not for what the worker wishes he were. The worker tries to understand where the client is at the moment and work from there.

Non-judgmental attitude. This precludes assigning guilt or innocence, and blame is regarded as outside the worker's function. The whole question of whether a person is worthy or unworthy of help is a quaint anomaly, though many workers continue to feel that moral judgments must be made.

Self-determination. This is one of the most difficult things to give a client. Workers who are asked for help must give help and advice, but just as surely every client has a right to reject help, to take advice or to reject it. The client has ownership of his or her problems. The concept of individualization and acceptance include a recognition of the individual's right to self-determination.

Confidentiality. Every client has the right to expect confidences to be kept.

The above principles must be upheld by the therapist; however, that does not mean the therapist will ignore his or her own feelings, or is not entitled to respect. Because of the strength of the male survivor's defenses, it is incumbent upon the therapist to maintain the principles, thereby utilizing the powerful change tool of role-modeling.

When therapists look for role models, especially in formulating a warm and empathetic approach to a client, the name of Carl Rogers usually surfaces. Roger's concept of unconditional positive regard serves to narrow the gap between client and therapist. Roger's Client-Centered Therapy requires that the therapist provide an atmosphere of unconditional positive regard so that the client can come to believe that his feelings are worthwhile and important. Survivors have a right to expect this in any therapeutic setting. The therapist must be not only warm and friendly, but also empathetic. He or she must use empathy to try to help the client articulate his feelings. It is not necessary to agree with

Roger's theory that persons who exist in an environment of unconditional positive regard will follow their own instincts for goodness and will become self-actualizing. It is only necessary that the therapist create a safe therapeutic environment through the use of ongoing warmth and empathy.

Whether a sexual-abuse survivor is male or female, the therapist will likely do his or her utmost to ensure social work principles are in place and a warm, empathetic setting is established. The intensity of male clients in relation to issues of anger and mistrust may dictate that establishing and maintaining a positive and trusting relationship will represent one of the most difficult challenges of any therapist–client situation. Patience and perseverance, along with a commitment to the social work principles and positive regard, may prove to be the difference in whether or not positive outcome is achieved.

Developmental Stages of Therapy

While establishing the relationship warrants special attention for male survivors, therapy does not stop there. It is always helpful in therapy to have at least some idea of what the future of a case may look like, and to that end I have developed the stages of therapy as they occurred with sexually abused men. Within the stages, anger, mistrust and meaninglessness will be very much in evidence. I have endeavored to expand on situations where repression is part of the process as it unfolds. There are four stages:

Stage 1	Engaging Strengths
Stage 2	Setting Goals
Stage 3	Removing the Symptoms
Stage 4	Maintaining the Change

Stage 1 Engaging Strengths

Men often attend therapy unsure of where the process will take them and unsure of their role and that of the therapist. They may be emotionally defensive and somewhat disorganized concerning agenda expectations. Many men may view therapy as a place people are expected to vent and therefore may unleash a verbal attack on the abuser, authorities, friends and family members. Such a common start to therapy really signals that the client feels he is expected to vent. Of more importance is the tone of venting, which allows the therapist to witness the degree of anger and rage that exists. On occasion, I have sat through as much as 30 minutes of uninterrupted venting as soon as the introductions were over. Such venting is accompanied by escalating anger, some of which has no doubt been suppressed. I usually avoid intervening at this point, for there is much information forthcoming, such as occasions where the client will angrily denounce authorities or therapists for thinking an abused man should be able to remember how he felt throughout the abusive events, or should remember all of the events.

Listening closely will indicate that the patterns shown by male clients point directly to repression. This fact might not surface should early intervention be targeted toward resolving anger. Male clients will normally vent toward the past but will return to their present situations without any prompting. Since the present is where we want to be for the purposes of solutions, there is no need to intervene. While this beginning to therapy may be uncomfortable, the principle stands that purposeful expression of feeling is a need and negative feelings are as important as positive.

Mistrust will appear in the first stage of therapy. To some survivors, acceptance and approval appear so unlikely that they defensively reject or depreciate the therapy by silently derogating the therapist and by reminding themselves that the setting is unreal and artificial. Given time, the male may verbally express his concern rather than keep silent. The chief concern in this instance is with intimacy and closeness.

Most clients I have treated informed me that they thought that, in therapy, they were expected to disclose their private thoughts and feelings to a total stranger. This process would be difficult enough at the best of times, and impossible for the abused male to achieve. Often resistance in the form of mistrust is deeply ingrained. Keep in mind that resistance is not usually conscious obstinacy, but more often stems from sources outside of awareness. At the early stage of therapy, concentration on the issue of mistrust in order to pursue solution would result in the client's slipping back into his habitual remoteness. Efforts to alter the pattern of mistrust during stage 1 would not only be unsuccessful but would assume crisis proportion, possibly ending in termination.

An enormously effective intervention at this stage is a common-sense approach to warmth and empathy. I say common-sense approach because the sexually abused male is sensitive to being patronized; therefore, compliments must be sincere. Statements such as "I understand how you feel" may be met with much hostility, for abused males may rightfully proclaim that nobody can ever imagine how they feel. The therapist must continue to validate, just as the client will continue to vent and possibly invite rejection.

Meaninglessness usually surfaces in stage 2 and need not be a concern during stage 1.

Unfortunately, it is difficult to measure success in therapy. I shall try to give an example of a successful stage 1 that occurred in my practice. I had seen a male survivor for three sessions and most of the content consisted of his venting about family and friends and their lack of understanding about his feelings and behavior. I simply listened intently and did not offer to intervene with therapeutic goals, nor did I mention solution-seeking. I did all I could to exhibit acceptance and made as many validations as possible. I saw the client as creative and resourceful in spite of his own efforts to sabotage his success. Later in therapy the client and I discussed this accepting approach in the early stages, and he stated that this approach really paid off. This became apparent at the end of the fourth session, when the client asked if he could make a further appointment. He had not voluntarily requested an appointment prior to this occasion. His reason for wanting to return for another session was "I don't know if counseling will help, but it's nice to come and talk to you about all this stuff." Such a statement is actually an indication of success in stage 1; the client is beginning the process of non-resistance. It was the beginning of an effective relationship.

Engaging strengths means having two people come together and do what they do best. I am not about to get caught up in the content of the stories of my clients. Instead, I observe process and patterns of interactions. My observations in early sessions with male survivors provided me with evidence of such strengths as determination, courage, assertiveness, sense of humor and resourcefulness, as these men vented their frustrations with life-long pain. I believe a few sessions of venting is not unreasonable, considering the years of emotional suffering these men have experienced.

The therapist engages in strengths by exhibiting his or her own qualities early in therapy. Persevering with positive regard requires patience and caring under difficult conditions. Warmth and empathy are essential. The therapist's experience with case-work may determine whether he or she is able to avoid the temptation to address content and defer solution work to a later stage of therapy. Engaging strengths should enable the therapist to gain a better understanding of the survivor's story and, at the same time, ensure that every opportunity is afforded the survivor to prepare for future sessions that will eventually focus on solutions.

Stage 2 Setting Goals

Many sexually abused men expect that negatives will follow positive experiences as they go through life. Therefore, the inevitable task of setting the agenda or goal-work may be met with much resistance. Such resistance would have as its base a strong sense of meaninglessness. It is not surprising that one who expects negatives always to follow positives would have a sense of meaninglessness; why would he not want to protect from positives if they will be followed by negatives? Since the client may be disorganized and resistant with regard to goal-work, the therapist must play a vital role in establishing how to proceed in this important area of therapy.

When we have a clear view of the facts, as established in stage 1, the next step is to construct a reasonable set of clinical goals. I cannot overemphasize the importance of setting clear and appropriate goals; in fact, it may be the most important step in therapy. The goals must be clear not only to the therapist but to clients as well. Goals must be tailored to the capacity and potential of the client. It is important that goals are achievable. Sexually abused men often enter therapy feeling defeated and demoralized; the last thing they need is another failure. The therapist represents the formulator of goals, yet must enlist the client as a collaborator—not an easy task. How do realistic goals materialize in spite of the difficulties mentioned? The answer can be found in setting the goals around the three major symptoms and not getting side-tracked by other issues.

Utilize the three major symptoms to form goals. Anger, mistrust and meaninglessness are present in most of the venting we witness in stage 1, so we are able to discuss these issues with the survivor. We then formulate these three symptoms into goals. As we have seen in previous chapters, male survivors are not inclined to deny or object to any of these symptoms and we are able to set goals that are realistic and achievable in a gradual fashion.

As an example of pulling these symptoms out of a conversation and eliciting the survivor's collaboration in setting goals, I recall one case where I was able to work with a client on his anger. He had described an event where he and his wife had engaged in one of their frequent conflicts. He had disciplined his son and felt justified in doing so. However, his wife disagreed with his actions and accused him of being too harsh and picking on the son. The client became very angry, and an argument ensued. This scenario turned out to be a frequent one in that family system. Once the client became angry, the whole focus of the issue changed from the son to a yelling match with hurtful accusations. Of course, at that point, there was little or no chance of resolving the conflict.

The key to using such a story to set goals around anger lies in the therapist's addressing the process and avoiding discussion of content. Dealing with content would result in the therapist's attempting to resolve the issue of the wife and son. The focus would be on the possibility of reaching some compromise about discipline that might end the frequent struggle. While this might seem to be a natural path to follow, it would result in missing the opportunity to address a much larger picture. The process, in this instance, can be seen in the client's getting angry and losing focus on the real issue of the conflict. This anger is a frequent pattern, as we saw in the chapter on anger, the secondary emotion. In my discussion with the client, he was finally able to articulate that his wife's acts of taking the son's side and questioning his own competence brought on feelings of rejection and hurt. Feelings were shifted to anger and the whole problem of conflict was never resolved. This process is indeed a larger issue than simply content.

The same kind of process thinking can bring forward issues of mistrust and meaninglessness. Those issues would then be added to the goal-work. In evaluations of therapy by my whole caseload of sexually abused males, there was overwhelming consensus that the formulation of goals around anger, mistrust and meaninglessness at this stage of therapy had a large influence on the ultimate positive outcome.

During the goal-setting stage, it is important that the therapist proceed with confidence in the fact that the appropriate approach is to work with the three major symptoms. There are at least two reasons why clients, in the end, were in favor of that approach. (1) No matter how highly functioning or emotionally strong the survivor may appear, there is much evidence that focusing on other symptoms may prove to be intolerable and result in early dropout. (2) Many clients reported a dramatic reduction or elimination of other symptoms upon recovery from anger, mistrust and meaninglessness.

Stage 3 Removing Symptoms

During preceding stages, much information has been exchanged between therapist and client. As I stated earlier, I prefer to inform the male survivor about the unconscious forces that dictate his feelings and behaviors. Usually, within stages 2 or 3 we discuss repression and how it relates to symptoms. There has been much evidence among my clients that a cognitive component (that is, knowledge and understanding) is essential; successful male survivor clients acquired either information or personal insight during the course of therapy.

However, intellectual insight alone is insufficient to create and maintain change. There must be an emotional component. Stage 3 is concerned with corrective emotional experience. The concept was introduced in 1946 by Franz Alexander. The basic principle of treatment is to expose the client in the present, under more favorable circumstances than in the past, to emotional situations that he could not handle in the past. The therapist helps the survivor tell which emotional reactions are appropriate and which are inappropriate. There must be systematic reality testing as well. The client proves to himself that he can indeed handle these situations.

The principle of corrective emotional experience is very much in evidence in chapters 2, 3 and 4. You will note that treatment issues surrounding the three major symptoms consist of a gradual exposure to new behavior in real-life situations. Because the steps are gradual and controlled, and with the concurrent therapeutic setting for support, the male survivor will experience a tolerable vulnerability rather than a crisis, which would result in relapse and an end to therapy.

To give success every opportunity to prevail, it is important that the first symptom we address is anger. In any multi-problem therapeutic situation where anger is present, it has been my experience that the client will repeat patterns of anger whenever intensity surfaces. For example, should the therapist and client be developing plans around a corrective emotional experience involving mistrust, the client may become angry if the situation becomes too difficult. Such anger would take attention away from the work around mistrust and it would be necessary to start all over again.

The removal of anger as a symptom requires a commitment to the treatment described in Chapter 2, and the fewer distractions the more probability of success within a reasonable period of time. As the client progresses toward removing anger, he will see certain treatment situations as having failed; however, in keeping with a solution focus, the therapist will be in a position to help the client recognize that some part of the corrective experience was successful. The focus will then be placed on expanding the part of the new experience that worked. This is a very important part of removing any symptom. In essence, the client will see the part of the corrective emotional experience that did not work. The therapist will see the part of the same experience that did work. The treatment will recommence with a view toward expanding the part that did work. While this treatment process is not easy, I have witnessed marvelous results as very angry men overcome their problem areas and begin to lead more productive lives without anger.

Mistrust requires the same dedication as anger to overcome it. The theme in mistrust treatment is to increase self-worth; this requires much goal-work in a behavioral model, and just as much commitment to recognizing resistance to success. The latter is probably the most difficult part of the treatment, as early messages of low self-worth will prove to be a formidable opponent when the client's worth as a human being becomes the center of attention. As discussed earlier, the focus of the treatment aimed at increasing self-worth would see symptoms of mistrust decrease as a feeling of self-worth increases. Again, perseverance and courage are the main requirements in advancing to positive outcome.

I usually leave meaninglessness until the last part of therapy. The reason for this is that it does not seem feasible to instill meaning into a life while anger and mistrust are outstanding symptoms. As I advanced in treatment issues with sexually abused men, I discovered that I had overlooked meaninglessness on numerous occasions in previous therapy. It occurred to me that meaninglessness could be misinterpreted as depression, lack of motivation, fear of success or apathy. Rather than make some sort of assessment to determine the existence of meaninglessness when dealing with male survivors, I make the assumption that this area of the client's life will require assistance. In any event, treatment for meaninglessness—learning how to immerse ourselves in life in a balanced way—can be of benefit to anyone.

As the therapist and client advance through corrective emotional experiences with the three major symptoms, it must be kept in mind that each venture into such an experience constitutes a critical incident for the survivor. While some negative affect (feelings) will be produced, the survivor should be profoundly impacted by positive affect (feelings) as the experience unfolds. Such an impact is likely to be threefold:

1. The client experiences strong positive emotions, which may be an unusual experience for him.

2. The feared catastrophe of the client's new response will not occur, namely, derision, rejection or engulfment.

3. The client discovers a previously unknown part of the self and thus is able to relate to others in a new way.

This stage of therapy represents much risk-taking by the client, as new experiences are planned and carried out. The survivor must both have a powerful experience and, through debriefings with the therapist, understand the implications of that emotional experience. That is the cognitive element, which has direct relevance to the here and now. I believe work in the here and now is essential to positive outcome, and the therapist's task is to direct the survivor to self-reflection. The more work in the here and now, the more increase in power and effectiveness in the therapeutic setting. The relationship between use of the here and now and use of the past will be discussed later in this chapter.

Stage 4 Maintaining the Change

The concept of maintaining positive change is of paramount importance, and constitutes a keystone upon which future healthy functioning rests. Facing and working through the three major symptoms enables the survivor to change and to employ his considerable potential constructively in later relationships and endeavors. The potential exists for relapse to occur should the survivor be exposed to critical incidents that can be associated with original causal experiences in the past. Stage 4 presents a safeguard against relapse when these critical incidents are experienced in future.

There are four main triggers for such critical incidents. Following are the triggers, with possible action plans to overcome them.

LOSS. Everyone will suffer loss during his lifetime, and such an event can trigger intense response. The threat to sexually abused men is that they may associate, unconsciously or otherwise, the present loss with enormous losses suffered in the past, whether these be childhood separation or abuse at the hands of a significant other. The issue of loss as a normal transition in life must be discussed, taking the view that we know what to do *when* loss occurs, not *if* loss occurs. This point in therapy would be a good time to review with the survivor a list of the strengths he has displayed in past successes. These strengths can be incorporated into a coping strategy to deal with potential losses. The process of grief must be normalized and the survivor may benefit from knowing that everyone grieves under certain conditions; indeed, stages of grief can be anticipated. The main goal, should loss occur, would be to allow the grieving process to take place and not to return to old defenses such as avoidance or suppression of emotions. There is a distinct benefit in establishing a support network of caring others.

BETRAYAL. The fact that a person may learn to love himself and overcome constant thoughts of mistrust does not guarantee that someone close will not take hurtful action against that person. Betrayal may present a formidable obstacle in future in that it represents a specific loss of trust. Association with the past may be strong, just as other losses may produce the same association. Anger and mistrust represent old coping mechanisms, and the survivor should look forward to developing new methods to deal with potential betrayals. One of the strategies I have found successful is to have the survivor remind himself that betrayal is the responsibility of the person doing the betraying, and so that person is given such responsibility. Put another way, betrayal says more abut the person betraying than it does about the person on the receiving end.

SELF-BLAME. For the male survivor, success and meaning have been elusive in the past. Feelings of aloneness and failure have been predominant. A pattern of self-blame has been established early in life whenever negative outcome is experienced. Negative outcome *will* occur, and care must be taken that the survivor does not resort to old patterns that would result in the view that he is different from others and destined to fail. Because of the strength of this pattern from repetition alone, it must be reiterated that negative does not necessarily follow positive. It is possible to overcome negatives and experience happiness again. Should a survivor note a recurrence of this pattern of self-blame, perhaps one or two visits back to the therapist would be in order.

INTIMACY. Where issues of intimacy are concerned, the threat of relapse may be considered as a lifelong risk. New romance or closeness with another may trigger a critical incident resulting in the need to withdraw. In the past, intimacy played a big part in the confusion of feelings, as discussed in previous chapters. Strong defenses against the potential for hurt may have enough force to regress the survivor to past unhealthy coping strategies. Everyone concerned in the therapeutic process must ensure that self-love is at a level sufficient to deal with vulnerability. Again, should self-love be in jeopardy, a visit with the therapist may be necessary to reinforce the survivor's sense of worth.

Together the client and therapist can develop plans to minimize a potential relapse for each individual case. The subject of maintaining recovery should be addressed, and goals should be set to help the client recognize critical incident triggers and take appropriate action. This is a far better approach than simply hoping all will go well in future. Sexually abused men can be retraumatized by events associated with the past and may need reinforcement of their strengths. Perhaps the leading prevention of relapse would be to leave the door open to further therapy which, in all likelihood, would be brief in nature.

Use of the Past

Irvin Yalom stated that the powerful and unconscious factors that influence human behavior are by no means limited to the past. The future is also a significant determinant of behavior. In addition to past and future, unconscious forces in the immediate present constantly influence our feelings and actions. Chapter 1 describes how the past may affect our behavior through pathways such as repression, which is only one of many possible defenses. The future is a no less powerful determinant of behavior, as we all have within us a sense of purpose, and of idealized self, and a series of goals toward which we strive. These factors, both conscious and unconscious, all arch into the future and profoundly influence our behavior. The knowledge of our isolation, our destiny and our ultimate death deeply influences our conduct and our inner experience. To cite only one example, a person may have a need to attack, which covers a layer of dependency wishes that he does not express lest he be rejected. We need not ask how he got to be so dependent. The past need not be part of the explanation of the need to attack; in fact the future (his anticipation of rejection) plays a central role in his interpretation.

One formidable problem with explanations based on the distant past is that they contain within them the seeds of "therapeutic despair." If we are so fully determined by the past, whence comes the ability to change? The past, moreover, no more determines the present and the future than it is determined by them. The real past exists for each of us only as we constitute it in the present against the horizon of the future. It is widely recognized in psychology that clients, even in prolonged therapy, recall only a minute fraction of their past experience and may selectively recall and synthesize the past so as to achieve consistency with their present view of themselves. In the same way that one alters one's self-image, one may reconstruct the past. Once one reconstructs the past, this new past can further influence one's appraisal of the present and the future.

If the most potent focus of therapy is the here and now, are we to take the view that the past plays no role at all in the therapeutic process? Not at all. The past is a frequent visitor to the inner private world of clients during the course of therapy. Often a full understanding of the developmental events that shaped the survivor's viewpoint can benefit the therapist and the survivor by providing fuller knowledge of the survivor and adding to acceptance. As an example, a man with an angry and mistrustful attitude may suddenly seem understandable once his story is known. As stated earlier, I use the past to explain unconscious forces and this explanation is well met by male survivors; these processes of the past are important. Discussions of future anticipation, both feared and desired, and of past and current experiences are an inextricable part of human discord and therefore constitute an inextricable part of therapy. But, as Yalom stated, "The past is the servant and not the master."

Disclosure of Sexual Abuse

The question of whether or not to disclose to others constitutes a crisis situation for the male survivor. Periodically, I will have clients ask me whether they should tell others about their abuse. In other cases, the abuse has already been reported, and occasionally criminal proceedings are underway or completed.

Disclosure represents a transition from an inner-self struggle to public attention. Often male survivors report rejection and a new set of problems if they choose to make the transition. It is particularly disturbing for me to witness men who disclose and subsequently experience more pain, resulting in withdrawal from others and, on occasion, suicide. Such experiences can only mean that certain segments of society are not supportive of sexually abused males (perhaps because of a lack of understanding) and that the survivor did not fully understand the implications and possible consequences of disclosure to others. One of the misconceptions I must address is the belief that disclosure would result in closure and thus hasten recovery. There is no evidence that this is the case; in fact, many clients state that disclosure represents the beginning of a new struggle, which now involves others. I would encourage any male who is contemplating disclosure to attempt to learn from the experiences of males who have disclosed.

A 29-year-old client told me the story of his disclosure. He anticipated support from others and relief from lifelong symptoms of anger. He engaged a lawyer and brought a civil case against the abuser, who happened to be a close friend of the family. Things went from bad to worse. The client's family attempted to have him resolve the issue with the abuser and forgive him, which meant dropping the lawsuit. Certain family members became more closed when communicating with the survivor and some friendships became more distant. Then the unexpected happened. The abuser was acquitted because of lack of evidence. The judge stated that he believed the plaintiff but could not find the defendant guilty because there were no witnesses, and certain people served as witnesses to vouch for the character of the abuser. The client informed me he was devastated and lapsed into a state of depression. He felt that he would not be able to recover from the experience, and contemplated suicide. Fortunately, there was a true friend among his family members and he was urged to attend therapy. Even more fortunate is the fact that he did recover, although the relationship with his parents remains damaged.

This case is an example of a negative outcome of disclosure for which the survivor was not prepared. I am sure that there are cases where positive outcome has been experienced, but the point is that male survivors contemplating disclosure should know the risks involved prior to making a decision. I am not advocating that disclosure should never be undertaken, for such action brings a much-needed public profile to sexually abused males. I am simply stating that the health and safety of the person who was abused is the foremost consideration.

In cases where a male survivor asks me whether or not he should disclose, I reply with a question of my own: "What difference would it make?" This question is a solution-based strategy for establishing a good decision. The survivor and I may explore the answer to this question. The ultimate decision becomes contingent upon the following: Should the difference represent a positive, disclosure could be an option. Should the difference represent a negative, disclosure should not take place. Should the difference be unpredictable, disclosure may be deferred until a more appropriate time.

In the end, the client has to deal with the consequences of disclosure; therefore, the decision is his to make. I do, however, take the position as a therapist that care should be taken to ensure the survivor knows the risks of disclosure and can handle whatever takes place afterward.

Summary

The therapeutic process is highlighted by a warm and empathetic relationship. Biestek's standards of social work and Roger's unconditional positive regard serve as guidelines for the therapist to persevere through initial sessions, which may prove difficult because of the anger and mistrust displayed by the survivor. The four stages of therapy represent the development of the client–therapist relationship and the removing of symptoms once goals have been established. Because of the behavioral nature of the goal-work, the client should work at his own pace to gain the full effects of a corrective emotional experience. The therapist serves as a facilitator and as means to a reality check as recovery progresses.

Plans for maintaining recovery are a key component to ensuring recovery is lasting. The main critical incidents that might lead to relapse—loss, betrayal, self-blame and intimacy—could be addressed as a preventative measure. Plans to deal with relapse triggers may be individualized to each survivor. Use of the past is meaningful in treating male survivors; however, the potent force behind change is the here and now. The past may be viewed as the servant and not the master.

Disclosure to others should be the choice of the survivor. The consequences of disclosure may not be predictable in every case, but the more information the survivor has about disclosure, the better he is able to assess his position on that issue.

The treatment of sexually abused men requires an approach that demands the courage and perseverance of the survivor and the therapist. Treatment issues differ from those that are successfully used for sexually abused women. I acknowledge that anger, mistrust and meaninglessness are not the only major symptoms displayed by male survivors, but these symptoms are more acceptable to the survivor in treatment than other symptoms that may cause overwhelming vulnerability and early dropout. It has been extremely gratifying for me to witness the recovery of the men who chose to work with me to develop an effective treatment model. I enjoyed their resourcefulness and courage. Of no less importance is the resourcefulness and courage of spouses and other immediate family members. The loyalty and dedication of certain spouses over the years has been more than impressive, and it is difficult to describe the reaction when the male survivor is able to accept the relationship without question. The work around improving treatment for male survivors has significance in that a recovered male has a chance to gain happiness and fulfillment. His spouse and children deserve nothing less for their own lives.

Throughout the progress of this book, I received much positive feedback from family members, which encouraged me to continue my work. In the end, I have learned much about competence and potential that exists within the character of the sexually abused male and the fact that hope should always prevail.

REFERENCES

Alexander, F and French, T. *Psychoanalytic Therapy: Principles and Application.* New York: Ronald Press, 1946.

Berg, Insoo Kim, and Miller, Scott D. *Working with the Problem Drinker.* New York/London: W.W. Norton, 1992, p.82.

Biestek, Felix P. *The Casework Relationship from Introduction to Social Work.* Homewood, Illinois: Dorsey Press, 1983, pp. 9-11.

Emily, Gordon. "Book of Readings" (university material).

Frankl, Victor. *Will to Meaning.* New York: World, 1969, p. 155.

Freud, Anna. *The Ego and the Mechanisms of Defence.* New York: Universities Press, 1946.

Jersild, Artjur T. *Child Psychology.* Englewood Cliffs, New Jersey: Prentice-Hall, Inc., 1960, pp. 257-258.

Jung, C.G. *Collected Works: The Practice of Psychotherapy,* Vol. XVI, New York, 1966, p. 83.

Kroeber, T.C. "The Coping Functions of the Ego Mechanisms", 1963 (university material).

Rogers, C.T. *Client Centered Therapy*. Boston: Houghton Mifflin, 1951, cited from *Psychology, The Science of Behaviour*, Boston: Allyn and Bacon Inc., 1984, pp. 703-704.

Yalom, Irvin D. *Existential Psychotherapy*. New York: Basic Books, 1931, 1980, pp. 423-424 and 483.

Yalom, Irvin D. *Group Psychotherapy*. New York: Basic Books, 1931, 1980, pp. 181 and 186.